AF211864

ALYNA CARON

ACNE SOLUTION

The Essential Guide On How to Cure Acne
Naturally, Learn Expert Tips on How to Get Rid
Acne and Have Clear Skin For Life

Descrierea CIP a Bibliotecii Naţionale a României
ALYNA CARON
    ACNE SOLUTION. The Essential Guide On How to Cure
Acne Naturally, Learn Expert Tips on How to Get Rid Acne
and Have Clear Skin For Life / Alyna Caron – Bucharest: Editura
My Ebook, 2021
    ISBN

ALYNA CARON

ACNE SOLUTION

**The Essential Guide On How to Cure Acne
Naturally, Learn Expert Tips on How to Get Rid
Acne and Have Clear Skin For Life**

My Ebook Publishing House
Bucharest, 2021

TABLE OF CONTENTS

CHAPTER 1

Educating Yourself about Acne

If you think acne affects only teenagers, then think again. It commonly strikes adults on a daily basis. It can be overwhelming to start noticing breakouts of pimples, blackheads, or zits all over your face and you might not know what to do first.

Before you do anything else, visit or call your local, trusted pharmacist. Licensed pharmacists are always knowledgeable about skin products and will know which products will bring acne relief and which ones won't. Most pharmacists are very willing to help. If you don't already know one, try your local WalMart.

While you are at WalMart, check out some of the available natural remedies and products they have displayed near the pharmacy. Many natural products claim to completely cure your acne. Any good drugstore will also have displays of various supplements claiming to help with acne relief.

Educate yourself on the different causes of acne and you may discover what is causing your own skin to break out. Acne research is lengthy and still ongoing so experts are not absolutely certain about the precise causes of acne. There are a few possible causes, however, that everyone seems to be in agreement on.

Medications

Some medications, such as steroids, barbiturates, and anti-seizure drugs, are thought to contribute to skin disorders. Don't stop taking your prescribed medications, though, before first checking with your physician to see if they could be causing your acne.

Emotional Stress

Increasing evidence suggests that stress may contribute to acne and other skin problems. If you are stressed, try developing an exercise program and following it regularly. Exercise is a proven stress-buster.

Chocolate

Chocolate has not yet been proven to cause acne. Many people insist that eating chocolate will make you break out in pimples but no amount of research has ever proven this theory to be true.

Cosmetics

Since acne is triggered by plugged or blocked pores, we can safely assume that make-up and other cosmetic products containing oil will contribute to acne. Even "safe" products (those that are hypoallergenic and oil-free) may contribute to blackheads or zits because they cover up the skin. Any cosmetic product applied to the skin has the potential to clog the pores and interfere with acne treatment.

Frequently Scrubbing your Face

Acne-prone skin should always be kept clean, but only mild products should be used to wash it gently. Many people are under the impression that they should scrub their skin using harsh soaps when they have acne but this only aggravates and worsens the condition.

Pollution

High humidity and other unnatural environmental conditions (i.e. smog, fog) can promote acne as well as other disorders. If skin is exposed to humid conditions for a prolonged period of time, swelling occurs (which blocks the pores, thereby contributing to acne).

Dietary habits

Many people notice that certain foods they eat cause their acne to flare up. Your dietary habits can certainly contribute to breakouts and you should note the products causing the most problems so that you can avoid them in the future.

Common food culprits thought to worsen acne include fats and dairy products. Diets rich in zinc should be beneficial if you have acne. Taking zinc supplements is one alternative you might consider for the relief or treatment of acne.

CHAPTER 2

The Causes and Best Treatments for Your Acne

No one in the world is immune to acne. It affects people from all walks of life and from any age category. Acne does not show preferential treatment to males, females, rich people, or poor ones. Because everyone's skin is different, they all have different contributing factors that cause their particular kind of acne.

The most important part of your acne treatment is understanding what skin type you are and the most effective acne treatment to use on it. If you have oily skin, you would not want to use cleansing products, moisturizing products, or cosmetics that contain oil.

You should buy products that are oil-free. On the other hand, if you have dry skin, you would not want to use the oil-free products because your skin could use a little extra oil.

Both oily and dry skin need to be moisturized daily. Just because skin has extra oil does not mean it doesn't need moisturizer. Plenty of good oil-free moisturizers are available to use on oily skin. Dry skin has its own specific problems and should be moisturized with a product made especially for dry skin.

Topical skin treatments are designed to keep pores from clogging while getting rid of excessive dirt and oil on the skin's surface, as well as acne-causing bacteria. Certain oral medications exist that will keep your body from producing so much oil. Prescription creams and ointments will help keep your breakouts dry and will even promote fast cell replacement in those areas of your acne-infected skin that need it. Other medical and natural remedies exist that help in the treatment of acne.

Before you understand how to develop the proper acne care skin treatment for your skin, you should try to understand what is causing the acne in the first place.

Causes of Acne

Acne has many causes and all of them aren't fully understood or substantiated yet. Here are some of the most common causes:

- Hormones play a major role in acne development. The early teen years bring many hormonal changes to the body and those changes often cause constant breakouts of pimples, pustules, and even cysts. The adult years bring changes, too, especially for women. Premenstrual and pre-menopausal difficulties cause breakouts in alarming numbers of women. Because of the excess oil produced during hormone-caused acne, products that help to eliminate and reduce oil will be most helpful for this type of acne.

- Stress is certainly a common factor to the development of acne. When the body becomes tense, it releases chemicals and hormones that eventually turn into toxins and waste that the body must expel. Some of these waste products will be excreted through the skin and will contribute to acne.

- Some people still believe that chocolate, sugar, and other foods can cause acne to form. Most experts deny that food has anything to do with acne's development but the subject is still widely debated and researched so we can't be absolutely certain that particular foods don't contribute to acne.

- Cosmetics and skin-care products can also contribute to acne if the products being used are not for the correct skin type. Using oily products on oily skin can certainly contribute to outbreaks so it is important to choose your personal care products very carefully when deciding on the best acne treatment for your skin.

Other factors, such as lifestyle and environment, can also affect your skin. The best things you can do for your skin is learn how to properly care for it, keep it hydrated, keep it moisturized, and try to eliminate the factors that are causing your skin to have acne.

CHAPTER 3

5 Simple Guidelines for
Your Successful Acne Skin Treatment

People with acne consider it to be an annoying problem, one that frustrates them to the point of hopelessness.

Acne skin treatment does take time once acne has developed, but the truth is, if acne hasn't already started, then it is fairly easy to prevent its occurrence. If it has started to appear, then following your prescribed acne treatment should bring positive results in a short period of time.

No matter what your predicament, you can have healthy skin if you will keep a few guidelines regarding proper skincare in mind.

Keep your skin clean

Perhaps the most important part of your daily skin care regime is keeping your skin clean. It should be washed twice daily, morning and night, with a mild hypoallergenic cleanser. In addition, it should be cleaned after any activity that causes you to sweat an abnormal amount, such as strenuous activity or exercise.

Of utmost importance is the type of cleanser you use on your skin. Scrubbing your skin with a harsh, abrasive soap will only make your acne worse. If you don't know of a good cleanser for your skin type, then consult your dermatologist for advice. Once you have washed your skin (gently), then rinse it and pat it dry.

If your hair is oily, like your skin, then it should be shampooed daily because oil from your hair can easily find its way to your face and cause problems.

Shave carefully

Shaving is a problem generally affecting only men. As far as choosing which type of razor to use (electric or safety), it depends upon which is the easiest and most comfortable to use. When using safety razors, the short blade should be the only one used on acne-prone skin. Before apply the shaving foam, the beard should first be softened using soap and water. Shave very carefully and lightly to avoid irritating the blemishes that might be present.

Keep your hands off of your face

Manipulating (squeezing or popping) the bumps on your face will only cause them to spread or form ugly acne scars. Keep your fingers completely off of your acne blemishes or you run the risk of interfering with your acne treatment.

Cosmetics

Check your make-up products to ensure that they are hypoallergenic and do not contain oil. If they do, or if they are old, you should toss them out and buy new products. Be sure to read the product labels to ensure that they don't contain ingredients that will conflict with your acne treatment. Until your treatment progress, it may be difficult to use foundation or other liquid make-up products on your skin.

In addition to checking your make-up, you should also look at the shampoo and conditioner you use on your hair. If they contain oil, acne could start appearing on your forehead. Make sure all hair products are non-comedogenic.

Stay out of the Sun

Even if you think tanned skin makes your blemishes look better, beware of exposing your skin to the sun, especially throughout your acne skin treatment period. Prolonged sun exposure will age your skin rapidly and put you at risk for skin cancer.

In addition to the harmful effects of the sun on your skin, the acne medication you are using can react negatively when exposed to the sun's rays, making you much more likely to get sunburned.

CHAPTER 4

5 Facts Regarding Acne Treatment

Just the mention of the word "acne" fills some people with dread. They envision having to spend long hours caring for their skin by scrubbing it, applying expensive creams to it, and avoiding the foods they most love to eat in order to prevent pimples from breaking out all over their faces.

The great news is that advances are being made in the treatment of acne and experts are discovering new ways to prevent and treat this dreaded skin condition. Some of the old wives' tales about acne have proven untrue and new information about how to get clear, beautiful skin is being uncovered daily.

Take a look at these 5 little-known facts regarding acne treatment and skin care:

1. To scrub or not?

Although experts once thought that scrubbing was necessary to get clean, pimple-free skin, they now know that scrubbing skin with harsh abrasives only serves to irritate and injure the skin. Because skin is delicate, it can easily become damaged, leaving it unable to act as a shield against harmful bacteria. So scrubbing your skin with or without abrasives must be avoided.

2. Can the sun make my skin beautiful?

Although the sun is capable of stopping bacteria in its tracks, it also harms your skin by drying it out and clogging your pores. Prolonged exposure (more than 15 minutes per day) to sunlight will not help you obtain beautiful skin and should be avoided.

3. Will cold air help clear my skin of acne?

Extremely cold weather damages the skin much the same way as sunlight does by drying it out and clogging the pores. Cold air should be avoided because it will interfere with any progress you are making towards clearing up your acne breakouts. The best temperature for maintaining beautiful, clear skin is between 70 and 80 degrees F.

4. Will swimming harm my skin?

Swimming is an excellent choice, both for your fitness level and your acne-prone skin. Swimming in an ozone-purified indoor swimming pool, with water that is approximately 75 to 85 degrees F, will cool down your irritated skin, reduce stress, and provide great exercise for your entire body.

5. How can I avoid coming into contact with the bacteria that causes acne?

The best way to prevent bacteria-causing acne and have pimple-free skin is to keep everything around you as clean as possible. Bacteria thrive in linens, towels, and washcloths so you must wash them each time you use them. Some natural

21

products that have been proven to cut down on bacteria are vinegar, essential oils, and tea tree oil, all of which can be used to wash your linens and undergarments.

Following these 5 steps will help you effectively fight and control your stubborn acne because you will learn to change your bad habits.

Changing your unhealthy habits will lead to a healthier lifestyle which will, in turn, lead to beautiful, clear, acne-free skin.

CHAPTER 5

Treating Acne the "Natural" way

Acne is a common skin disorder involving the sebaceous glands of the face, back, and neck. Most people are affected by acne at some point in their lives and suffer with the resulting pimples, zits, blackheads, and cysts.

Sebaceous glands work to expel excess oil from the skin. Invariably, they are going to clog up from time to time and the resulting accumulation of oil can cause acne, as well as other skin conditions. Acne vulgaris is the most commonly experienced condition and affects primarily adolescents.

Many factors contribute to acne vulgaris and include nutritional imbalances, allergens, emotional stress, liver abnormalities, heredity, excessively oily skin, certain medications, and hormones.

Another contributing factor to acne is an overabundance of toxins and poisons in the body. The body uses the liver and kidneys to rid itself of these dangerous substances. If the body contains more impurities than those organs can effectively manage, the skin takes over by sweating out the substances.

All of these processes working at the same time upset the natural healing capacity of the body and create various skin conditions, causing pimples and zits to form.

There are many natural products available that will effectively treat acne. Listed below are several of the best and most well tolerated alternative methods for eliminating the effects of acne.

Keep in mind, however, that some of these methods may have to be repeated over the course of 2 to 4 weeks before any lasting results are noticed.

- Pat white vinegar (distilled and diluted if necessary) on areas of the skin affected by acne. Allow it to stay on skin for up to 10 minutes, and then rinse gently with cool water.

- Use Echinacea daily to improve immunity.

- Take Oregon grape daily to guard against acne-producing bacteria.

- Apply lemon juice to areas of the face affected by pimples, zits and other skin conditions. Let the juice stay on the face for up to 10 minutes, then rinse off with cool water. Other citrus juices may be used and diluted if they cause stinging sensations. This solution will work as a natural exfoliate by rubbing off dead skin tissue.

- Use dandelion or red clover daily to clear the liver of toxins.

- Use Natures Sunshine's Ayurvedic Skin Detox to remove toxins from the liver.

- Using Vitamin A supplements will help severe acne. Consult your physician to determine the correct dosage because overly large amounts can be toxic.

- Take Zinc supplements to encourage tissue repair and prevent scarring of the skin.

- Try Alternative Homeopathic remedies to dry pimples and heal damaged tissues.

- Follow a well-balanced diet and take vitamin and mineral supplements to prevent nutritional deficiencies. Keeping your body healthy will encourage natural healing of your tissues.

- Drink plenty of water daily to flush out toxins and to keep the body hydrated.

CHAPTER 6

Common Acne Myths

People continue to believe old wives' tales about the causes of acne, even though experts have now disproved many of the myths. We will attempt to reveal the truth about some of those die-hard myths and set your mind at ease so that you can move forward in your quest for clear, acne-free, beautiful skin.

Myth: Only dirty people have acne

Fact: Acne is not caused by poor hygiene but by hormonal changes taking place within the body. Sometimes the sebaceous glands (responsible for moistening our skin) become overrun with oil and block nearby follicles. This causes clogged pores, which turns into acne characterized by pimples, zits, pustules, and even cysts.

The truth is that consistent scrubbing and washing the skin can make your acne problem much worse. The proper skin care routine involves washing your skin gently and patting it dry (not rubbing it).

Myth: People with acne are not eating the correct foods

Fact: Experts now know that there is no connection between the foods you eat and the development of acne.

The myths claiming that chocolate and other fattening foods cause acne are completely erroneous. On the other hand, you do need to practice proper nutrition so that your overall health will be great.

Myth: Stress causes acne

Fact: Stress itself does not cause acne, although it can develop as a side effect when taking medications prescribed to help you cope with stress. If you take this type of medication and are noticing acne symptoms, such as pimples, zits, or pustules, consult with your physician to determine if the medication might be contributing to your skin condition. One word of caution: although stress will not cause acne, it can make the condition worse if you already have it.

Myth: Acne is purely cosmetic

Fact: Acne does change your looks but it can also pose a threat to your mental health. Serious acne problems, often characterized by cystic nodules and persistent eruptions, can lead to severe acne, causing permanent scars to form.

This sometimes affects people psychologically by altering the image they have of themselves. Many people develop problems with their self-esteem and become frustrated and depressed.

Myth: Acne is incurable

Fact: Acne can be completely cleared up by using the many products available and finding the correct treatment specific to your needs.

Your dermatologist can help you find the best method to treat your acne and will be able to determine which type of acne you have, whether it is acne vulgaris, cystic acne, nodular acne, or even rosacea. There are good, effective treatments and medications available (including Accutane, Retin-A, & many others) to help clear up even the most persistent problems. Before you know it, you will reveal the beautiful skin you were always meant to have.

CHAPTER 7

Using your Makeup Creatively to Conceal Acne

You finally took that important step by visiting your dermatologist and starting acne treatment earlier this week! Your skin will soon become clear, beautiful, and acne-free.

Congratulations! Did you say that you had an important meeting to attend tomorrow and you needed your skin cleared up by then? Well, your acne may not clear itself that quickly but there are some tips you can use in order to look your best at your meeting.

Using makeup creatively will enable you to conceal your acne temporarily but you must adhere to a few basic rules. Do keep in mind that this is only a cover-up, not a cure.

The basic essentials needed for your acne cover-up kit

Your most important acne cover-up tools will be concealer, foundation, and powder. Buy only brand name, trusted products from reputable stores. Choose oil-free, hypoallergenic products matching your skin color.

Read the product labels thoroughly to ensure that you aren't buying products loaded with oil that will halt your newly started acne treatment in its tracks. If you decide to try a new brand, test it out before using it by dabbing a little bit under your jaw line. If your skin is going to react negatively, it will do so within the hour.

Before starting the cover-up

Before you start the acne cover-up process, gently wash your face and neck with your usual cleansing product and then pat dry. Use your new acne treatment medication next by applying it according to the instructions. Allow this to dry completely.

The main event

Now you can start the cover-up process. Dab small amounts of concealer directly on red or darkened splotches of your face and neck that were caused by acne blemishes. Use a throwaway makeup sponge to blend the concealer into your skin.

Don't overdo this step because too much concealer will look awful once it dries. Apply it very lightly.

Now, dab small amounts of foundation on your skin, blending with the sponge. Reapply to areas that seem to need a little more coverage but, again, don't overdo, because too much makeup will draw attention to your acne-scarred skin.

Your final step is to apply a very light layer of powder, using a soft makeup brush. Always use oil-free powder with the softest brush you can find to avoid irritating your acne-troubled skin. The powder will absorb any shine left behind by your makeup and will also give your face that "finished" appearance.

Be certain to dispose of the makeup sponges you used during your cover-up. They will retain oil from your face and should be thrown out to avoid transferring that same oil to your face tomorrow.

Before going to sleep

Always wash your face before going to bed each night. Your skin needs that time to breathe and your acne does not need to have makeup coating it because additional blemishes may result. Apply your acne treatment again (according to instructions).

CHAPTER 8

Repairing Acne Scars

Acne, a common skin disorder that people spend millions of dollars trying to heal, generally affects 80% of our youth and 5% of our adult population. Young people, who are the ones most affected, spend hours agonizing over the ravaging effects acne causes to their skin.

At their young age, they are beset with social problems and popularity issues. The scars left by their battles with acne are damaging to their egos and self-esteem. Billions of dollars have been spent researching acne, acne scarring, and scar solutions.

There are three classifications of acne scars, Icepick, Boxcar, and Rolling. The duration of the scars also cause them to be broken down into two other groups, early or permanent.

Topical medications work well on early scars but surgical intervention is often needed for permanent scarring.

Combinations of treatments are sometimes used for both types, depending on their severity. Along with the available topical medications, skin resurfacing procedures and surgical procedures are used, as well, for the most severe scars.

Surgical procedures are expensive treatment options and there are both advantages and disadvantages to this type of acne scar solution. Before utilizing surgery, physicians will evaluate the patient's age, gender, history of medical problems, skin type, and scar type, among other things.

Sometimes, collagen or other injections can be used to raise the scar to skin level. These injections are called dermal fillers.

The "punch excision" procedure is frequently used by dermatologists when treating icepick or boxcar scars. This procedure involves slitting the skin with a special tool, and stitching the edges of the skin together. This forms a new scar that heals with clearer looking skin. There is also a variation of this procedure, called "punch excision with skin graft replacement."

It is much the same as the original procedure except for the skin being sewn together. It is, instead, skin-grafted to repair the scarring.

Subcutaneous Incision is yet another procedure but is used primarily on rolling scars. In this procedure, a needle is inserted into the skin and cuts the scar tissue. The skin bruises greatly during this procedure but clears up in about 1 week.

Laser resurfacing burns the topmost layer of skin, lowering it to the original skin level.

When you look at all these procedures used to treat scars, it is obvious that prevention is better than the cure.

To prevent scars from forming, try avoiding the sun, using alpha hydroxyl acids, exercising regularly, and maintaining good dietary habits. You might just save yourself a lot of unnecessary expense and humiliation.

CHAPTER 9

Treating Acne Scars – Can Acne Scars Be Removed?

Scars are indications that the body has repaired itself in one way or another, either due to injury or infection. Once these events occur, white blood cells from the body accumulate at the site to fight further infection and repair the damage that has taken place.

Once that process is complete, scars often form. This process can be compared to a seam being sewn into a piece of torn fabric. The skin (or seam) will never be quite as smooth as it was before the damage.

There are different types of acne scars and different degrees of each type. Some people may develop worse scars than others, depending on their individual tendencies.

Types of acne scars

There are two different types of scars caused by acne. The first type, depressed scarring, is caused by tissue loss and the second type, keloids, is caused by tissue formation.

1) Depressed Scarring

This type of scar is caused by the dermis being attacked by toxins escaping the skin. Once a cyst ruptures, it expels pus, oil, bacteria, and other poisons into the surrounding areas.

White blood cells rush to the site of infection to repair the skin and, in the process, valuable collagen is lost, causing skin recesses or depressions. The skin above the injury will then develop scars most commonly called ice pick scars. Other scar types are soft, mascular, and fibrotic.

2) Keloids

This type of scarring results from fibroblasts being triggered by the body during the repair process. Once collagen starts decreasing, the fibroblasts produce excessive collagen, resulting in tissues called keloids. They usually form on the male body and are sometimes called hypertrophic scars.

Treating the scars of acne

Consult your dermatologist about the best treatment for your individual scars. Be prepared to discuss your feelings about the scarring, the cost of treatment, and what you want the end result of the treatment to be. The physician will need to consult with you regarding the severity and location of the scars, as well as what type of treatments are available.

Commonly requested scar treatments include laser, collagen, and dermabrasion. Skin surgery and/or grafting are also considerations if the scars run deep. Keloids are sometimes left alone if the physician feels that treatment will cause other keloids to form.

In this event, keloids can sometimes be effectively remedied by using steroid injections.

CHAPTER 10

Vitamins, Minerals, and other
Supplements that Eliminate Acne

Many supplements exist that will help speed up the success of your acne treatment. It is well known that taking certain vitamins, minerals, or other types of supplements will help to eliminate skin disorders. We are listing some of the most effective ones to use when fighting acne.

1. Vitamins

- 50,000 IU of water-soluble Vitamin A should be taken right before eating. Don't take more than this amount before first getting your physician's approval because too much Vitamin A can be toxic. If you start experiencing unwanted symptoms with this dosage, then decrease it to 25,000 IU.

- 500-1000 mg of Vitamin B5, or pantothenic acid, should be taken daily

- 25-150 mg of Vitamin B6 should be taken daily (Vitamin B6 should be one of the vitamins in a B complex vitamin).

- 1000 mg of buffered Vitamin C should be taken three times daily.

- 400 IU of Vitamin E should be taken twice daily and must be taken before eating.

2. Minerals

- One tablet of Calcium Hydroxyapatite Complex should be taken 3 times daily after every meal.

- 200-500 micrograms of Chromium should be taken daily.

- 25-60 mg of Zinc Gluconate should be taken once daily. Never exceed 100 mg unless you get your physician's approval. Zinc is, by far, the most important mineral to take in your quest for freedom from acne because it reduces DHT, the male sex hormone that can cause acne if there is an excessive amount of it in the body.

3. Oxygen Elements Plus

Oxygen Elements Plus is a nutrient that, with proper use, will add 10 to 20% more oxygen to your blood. Aside from the beneficial oxygen, this product also contains other useful minerals and nutrients.

Acid, waste products, and pathogens serve to use up much of the oxygen you receive. The amount left behind is what your body must use for the rest of its needs. Because you need more oxygen than is readily available, Oxygen Elements Plus is a great product to help you get it. Your skin needs oxygen to stay clean and bacteria-free. More oxygen may result in you having clear, acne-free skin.

4. Other Special Supplements

Six special supplements exist, in addition to Oxygen Elements Plus, that might clear your acne, as well as improve your level of health and immunity to infections.

- Mineral Electrolytes
- Digestive Enzymes
- Lecithin

- Chlorophyll
- Systemic Enzymes
- Flax Seed Oil

These supplements should be used according to the directions on their individual labels.

It is important to discontinue using any of the supplements we have mentioned here (especially the ones with high dosages) once your acne is under control.

Once things get back to normal, you should continue whatever supplementation program you were originally using. Prolonged use of supplements in high dosages can sometimes cause a chemical imbalance in your body and can be harmful to your health.

Printed by Libri Plureos GmbH in Hamburg, Germany